My Alzheimer's Diary

A Memoir of Alzheimer's Diagnosis

OTHER BOOKS BY RAYNETTA MANEES

All For Love (Book 1 of the SuperStar Series)

All For Love: The SuperStar (Book 2 of the SuperStar Series)

Fantasy

Follow Your Heart

Wishing On A Star

Heart Of The Matter

All The Way Home)

[All The Way Home is a novella originally published in the "A Mother's Touch" Anthology. It is now available in a stand-alone edition.]

My Alzheimer's Diary:
A Memoir Of Alzheimer's Diagnosis
By
Raynetta Manees

eBook ISBN: 978-0-9855324-5-1
paperback ISBN: 978-1-7321342-3-2

Please visit
Raynetta Manees Books on Amazon.com   or
Raynetta Manees Books on Barnes and Noble.Com
(Bn.Com)
for a FULL LIST of the author's books

Please visit the author's personal website
http://www.RManees.com/ for additional author
information and author appearances

Dedication

This book is lovingly dedicated to my mother, the late Lebertis Knight Manees Wright, and my brother, the late Roland Knight. Alzheimer's disease took them both of away from us far too soon.

Acknowledgments

My family steadfastly stood by me during the creation and promotion of this journal. And even more importantly, they stood by me during the period outlined in this book.

My love and undying thanks to my daughter, Tiffani Young, my granddaughter, Zayna Ray'lon Hurd, and my grandson, Jeffrey Young, Jr. (AKA Jellybean).

Preface

When I began "My Alzheimer's Diary" I already knew quite a bit about Alzheimer's. It had attacked three generations of my family.

"More than half of Americans [54%] report that they have been touched by someone (living or deceased) who has Alzheimer's disease, and roughly a third of Americans are worried about getting Alzheimer's."[1]

With over half the country personally touched by Alzheimer's, interest in the disease is skyrocketing.

Alzheimer's had a noteworthy impact on the 2015 Oscar Awards. "Rhinestone Cowboy" country superstar Glen Campbell won an Oscar for his song "I'm Not Gonna Miss You." The song was written by Campbell (with Julian Raymond) for his family after his 2011 Alzheimer's diagnosis. This was Campbell's first Oscar nomination, but, due to his deteriorating health, he was unable to attend the Oscars. His writing partner said that, sadly, Campbell didn't understand their nomination.[2]

Also that night, actress Julianne Moore won the Best Actress Oscar for her performance in "Still Alice." Moore plays a university professor diagnosed with early onset Alzheimer's disease.

Although several members of my family have developed Alzheimer's, I was not directly involved in these diagnoses of the disease. I knew a lot about the care of Alzheimer's patients, but very little about what happens before.

Now it was my turn. It was suspected that I had Alzheimer's. During this stressful time, I did a lot of research on Alzheimer's disease. There was plentiful information defining Alzheimer's, or giving the warning signs of Alzheimer's, or how to cope, as either a patient or caregiver, once Alzheimer's was confirmed.

But to my dismay, I found there was far less information about the *process* of diagnosis. You think you may have Alzheimer's. What's next? Your first stop would, of course, be your family doctor, but what happens then?

The majority of this book is a diary: "A record with discrete entries arranged by date reporting on what has happened over the course of a day or other period...It is generally written not with the intention of being published as it stands, but for the author's own use."[3]

That is exactly how this book came into being. It was written for my own use, to help me get through a difficult, confusing, and frightful time.

I have been a published author since 1996. Until now my published work has been exclusively fiction, primarily novels. As a novelist, I naturally turned to writing as a means of managing—and at times restraining—my anxiety. So this diary was not initially intended for publication.

But I began to think about the family I've lost to Alzheimer's, and in time I came to feel it wasn't right for me to keep this story to myself. I owed it to them to tell it.

The bulk of this journal was written on the dates indicated. At points I have inserted brackets with additional information needed for the reader's comprehension.

Introduction

Even before December 18, 2011, I was well acquainted with Alzheimer's disease due to its devastating effects on my family. I was familiar with the disease and its treatments. And I knew only too well about its effects, having watched it slowly but surely whittle away at the minds of people I loved.

On December 18, 2011, my personal journey with Alzheimer's began. It started with a car accident.

It was a Sunday evening. I was driving to my neighborhood post office to mail a Christmas gift. My granddaughter, Zayna, was in the car with me. She was looking down, staring at her cell phone, texting or something or another, as teenagers seem to incessantly do.

This was the last of several errands. I remember that as I drove along I was glad to finally finish my errands and return home, there being gifts to wrap and several other Christmassy details to be finalized.

In what seemed like the next moment I heard my granddaughter scream, "Grandma!" I looked up to see headlights coming directly at me. I was across the center line, on the wrong side of the street! Instinctively I gave the steering wheel a sharp turn, in an attempt to avoid a collision. The driver heading towards me did the same, in the opposite direction. As a result, we were able to avoid a full frontal head on collision. We almost avoided a collision altogether, but not quite. My front left fender clipped the oncoming car's front left fender.

Fortunately, no one was injured, and the damage to both cars was minor. We called the police; a policeman came and took a report. The other driver did not wish to exchange insurance information. He said his car sustained almost no damage at all.

In my 40 years of driving, this was my third accident, but the only one that had been my fault. I lucked up; the police officer who took the report did not issue me a ticket. I was also lucky in that the other driver did not wish to report his damage to my insurance company. (I thought this rather strange, but I guess he had his reasons.)

I was even fortunate in my dealings with my insurance company. Although I openly admitted to them the accident was totally my fault, they elected not to raise my insurance rates since I had been such a loyal customer and safe driver for such a long time.

I put my car in the dealership for repair, got the rental car my insurance provided, and four days later I had my car back, repaired and looking like new.

That was the end of it—or so I thought. Little did I know, it was just the beginning.

Thursday, May 31, 2012

This has been one hell of a day. Since I'm having so much
trouble wrapping my head around this, and since I can't
sleep anyway, I've decided to come into my office and do
what I so often do when I'm hashing something out in my
mind—write it down.

When Tiffani [my adult daughter, Zayna's mother] called
me this afternoon and told me she needed to talk to me, I
knew it was a matter of some importance. Tiffani and I
talk on the phone at length all the time. So the fact that she
wanted to come over and talk to me in person let me know
right away it wasn't a run-of-the-mill issue.

Another tip off was that she wouldn't tell me what she
wanted to talk about. When I asked her she said, "I'd rather
talk to you about it in person." Although I had no idea
what it could be, I assumed the matter concerned one of my
grandchildren, or my daughter herself.

When Tiffani got here, I made a pot of coffee since we both
drink too much of the stuff. We sat down at my kitchen
table for our discussion.

"Okay," I said, "What up? What's the big emergency?"
She didn't smile. This immediately set off alarm bells in
my head. Whatever the problem was, it had to be
something serious. I knew my child and I knew from her
demeanor that something was amiss.

She still hadn't spoken. She just sat there, looking down
into her coffee cup.

"All right, Tiff," I finally said, "I can tell you've got
something major on your mind. I'm certain the disasters

I'm imagining are ten times worse than the real problem. So why don't you put me out of my misery and just tell me what this is all about." I paused a moment. "Is something wrong with one of the kids?"

She looked up then. "No, Mama," she quietly answered.

"Is something up with Jeff?" [Her husband]

"No, Mama," she repeated.

"Okay, we've now narrowed the subject matter substantially. So it's got to be something going on with you. Right?"

She slowly looked up at me, and a bolt of fear ran down my spine. I could tell whatever it was was difficult for her to say. Tiffani had experienced some rather serious health problems in the past, and at this is point my first thought was, *Oh, God, no. Please don't let anything be seriously wrong with her.*

"No, Mama," she said for the third time. "There's nothing wrong with me. But I think something may be wrong with you."

I could not have been more surprised. "*Me?* Honey, nothing's wrong with me. What are you talking about?"

Again she hesitated, and then finally said, "Mama, I've been thinking about this for a while. Trying to figure out what I should do. Trying to figure out if there really was a problem. I finally decided that there was and that I had to do something about it."

Now I was totally befuddled. "What in the world are you talking about? You've been worried about me for months? Why?"

She took a deep breath. "Mama, I think you might have Alzheimer's."

The world tilted. For a second it felt like I had physically lost my balance, and was about to tumble out of my chair. But I composed myself, and took a sip of coffee before I asked, "Why in the hell do you think I have Alzheimer's?"

"Mama, I didn't say you had Alzheimer's, but from the way you've been acting lately, I think it's sure a possibility."

"*What* 'way I've been acting lately?' What have I done to make you think that?"

"Well, you know how often you've been losing things lately. You're always telling me that you're looking for something in the house that you can't find. And you also know how you mix up peoples' names sometimes."

"Yes dear, I know all that. But I'm in my sixties now. Forgetting things happens naturally to a lot of people my age. I have to admit, for a while there I was becoming a little concerned about 'The Big A' myself, especially since it seems to run in our family.

"But I sat down and researched it on the Internet. And I found out what I just told you: some memory loss and that type of forgetfulness are very common and very natural for people as they grow older. I love you for worrying about me, honey, but there's nothing to worry about."

But rather than looking relieved, she looked more upset than ever. "But that's not the only thing, Mom. Remember about three months ago when I was looking for a house? I called you to come over and check out a house I was considering. I called because the house was so close to you that you could run by in a matter of minutes."

"Yes, of course, I remember. What has that got to do with this?"

"Don't you remember what happened that day, Mama? You should have been able to get from here to where I was in ten minutes or so, but it took you more like half an hour. I had to call your cell twice to ask where you were."

"I know, but as I told you, I got lost. You know how these subdivisions are with cul-de-sacs and stupid dead end streets. I just had a little trouble finding the place."

"Mama, you've lived in this house for 16 years. You know the neighborhood like the back of your hand. There was absolutely no reason for you to get lost going from this point A to that point B."

"Yes dear I know, but..."

"Don't you remember what happened with Momo? [Momo was my mother, Tiffani's grandmother.] She suddenly started getting lost while driving around. And you know that other thing that she used to do, mixing up peoples' names. Sometimes she would look me dead in the face but still call me *your* name. You've been doing that mixing up names thing for quite a while now."

I had to really think about that one. She did have a point. I had forgotten about how my mother had started to get lost when driving. In fact, it rapidly got to the point where we didn't want her to drive at all anymore.

"Well, I guess I can see your anxiety about it. I mean, I have to admit there are certain similarities. And I appreciate your concern, honey, I really do. But I don't think…"

"Mom, I made an appointment to go see Dr. T." [Dr. T. is our long-time family doctor. We all see him, my daughter, my son-in-law, both my grandchildren, and myself.]

"I *know* you're not about to tell me you called and made an appointment for me with Dr. T. without my permission?" That I did not like one bit.

"No, Mama. I made an appointment with him for myself. I didn't want to discuss this situation over the phone. I wanted to talk to him face-to-face. So when I got there I told him the problem wasn't with me, it was with you. He said that although I was your daughter, he, of course, could not discuss your medical history with me without your permission. Then he said, "But there's nothing saying I can't *listen*.""

This really threw me off my stride. "So what did you tell him?"

"I told him about your getting lost. I told him about that car accident you had a few months ago. I told him how you've been losing things around the house, not able to remember where you put them. And Mama, you've been talking weird at times the last couple of months."

"Weird? What do you mean weird?"

"You've been repeating yourself. At times when we are talking you tell me something and 15 minutes later, you tell me the same thing. And you're mixing your words up a lot, which is really unusual for you. You say one word when I know that you really meant to say another. A couple weeks ago you called to tell me you had found the earring I lost."

"So?"

"So what you said to me was, 'Honey, I found the earning you lost."

"I did?"

"You sure did. And what concerns me most about it is that you didn't seem to realize what you had said. You didn't seem to realize that you had used the wrong word. Mom, you're a professional writer, an author. You've got a vocabulary that would probably wrap around the moon a few times. When *you* start stumbling over words and using words inappropriately it's cause for alarm."

It took me a moment to digest all that. Finally, I said, "And you told all this to Dr. T.?" She nodded. "Well, what did he say?"

"He was quite concerned when I told him how you were acting and how you were talking. I also told him that your grandmother, your mother, and your brother all had Alzheimer's. And that I read somewhere they found out there is a strain of Alzheimer's that is most likely hereditary.

"He said you need to make an appointment and come in to see him as soon as possible. He told me to tell you that, so that's what I'm doing."

So there it was. I really hadn't realized that I was doing some of the things she mentioned, and I guess I didn't recognize the significance of the problems I had noted myself. Now I'm wondering—did I really not notice those things or was it that I didn't *want* to notice them?

Friday, June 1, 2012

I called today and made an appointment with Dr.T for Tuesday, June 5th.

I don't really remember when I first worried about getting Alzheimer's. With our family history, I suppose it was inevitable that I contemplate having it myself one day.

I don't recall *when* it was, but I do remember *why* I first thought about developing Alzheimer's myself. It was when I started calling people by other peoples' names. For instance, I might call my daughter Tiffani "Marlowe." Marlowe is my niece, my sister's daughter. Or I might be referring to my friend Helen, but instead say the name of my friend Linda.

I had forgotten this was the first sign we had that something was wrong with my mother. As Tiffani reminded me, Mama had started doing that, and, now that I think about it, she started doing it when she was just about the age I am now.

Mama was an extremely kind and loving person, but she was also intensely determined and self-reliant as well. She was born in another time, a time when most families had only one car, and the husband did all the driving. Mama had stopped working when I was born, and from that time on was a housewife.

She had never learned to drive or gotten a driver's license throughout my childhood. But one day, when I was in college and my younger sister still in high school, for some reason Mama decided she wanted to drive. I already had a driver's license, so between my step-father (who wasn't too crazy about the idea) and me, we taught her to drive. She got her first driver's license when she was in her early fifties.

That's how she was. She'd think long and hard about doing something, but once she made up her mind, she did it, come hell or high water. And she never had any doubts about her ability to accomplish anything she set out to do.

When she started mixing up names, it became sort of a family joke. We teased her about it, and she'd laugh right along with us. Most people knew nothing about Alzheimer's then.

But Mama had Alzheimer's. My grandmother, her mother, had Alzheimer's. My older brother has Alzheimer's. [My brother passed away in 2014].

I'll never forget the last time my mother visited my grandmother, who lived in another state, 1,000 miles away. When Mama came home and we were discussing her visit, she suddenly started to cry. She was crying because her own mother did not recognize her. She said my grandmother, who was in bed, looked up at her, and asked, "Who are you?"

Mama had known ahead of time that my grandma had Alzheimer's, but she had not seen my grandma in years and had not experienced first-hand how just bad it had gotten. Mama said it hurt her to her very soul to have her own mother look at her and not know who she was.

I know how that feels—now. My mother passed away a little less than a year ago [in 2011]. Her Alzheimer's had gotten really bad in the years just prior to her death.

There were times when Mama would be in the past. She'd look at me and say, "Raynetta, you better hurry or you'll be late for school. Don't forget to get your lunch bag out of the fridge."

Or she'd start talking about her husband, my step-father. She'd say "I'd better hurry to get dinner started. Daddy will be home soon." My stepfather died in 1996.

Most of the time she recognized me, but there were times she didn't. And that hurts. No matter how many times it happens, you never get used to it and it never stops hurting.

I'm terrified that one day I'll look at my daughter and not know who she is.

Tuesday, June 5, 2012

I'm so glad Dr.T. is my doctor. Dr. T. knows his stuff
medically and he really cares about his patients. He's not
the type doctor to just shove a pill at you. I know.

A few years back I was having some numbness on the side
of one thigh when I woke up. He told me that frequently
happened to women as we age, and all I needed was a small
dose of quinine. At the end of the appointment I was
expecting to get a new prescription, but instead, he said,
"Oh, you don't need a pill for this. Just get yourself some
tonic water and drink half a glass before you go to bed.
That will give you all the quinine you need." That's what I
did. It took care of the problem just fine.

I've been seeing Dr. T. so long now that I've lost track of
exactly when he started treating me. It's got to be at least
ten years, probably longer.

Dr. T. has always been easy to talk to, and for that difficult
a conversation, a doctor that's easy to talk to is exactly
what's needed. When I went in this morning he greeted me
with the stink eye and asked why it took Tiffani coming to
talk to him for me to come in. Why hadn't I come in to see
him about my situation on my own?

I explained that I just thought these things were happening
naturally because I was getting older and that I really hadn't
been concerned.

But he said he *was*, with Alzheimer's disease being so
prevalent in my family. He also told me studies have
shown people with my medical conditions, diabetes for
one, were at higher risk to develop Alzheimer's.

Although Tiffani had already given him a pretty good run down on my circumstances, he asked me to go over this information again. He frowned when I told him about the car accident in December, saying, "You never told me about that."

He proceeded to ask me a series of questions and then told me he was relatively sure my symptoms were caused by either the early stages of Alzheimer's or by sleep apnea.

He ordered sleep apnea testing for me, which he said might take a while to schedule. But he felt it was imperative I see a specialist immediately to be evaluated for Alzheimer's. If I did have Alzheimer's it was important that I start the indicated medication as soon as possible.

He wrote up a referral for me to a neurologist in our health care system and gave me the number to call to schedule an appointment. He also did a referral to our system's sleep clinic. He told me they would call me to schedule my sleep apnea screening, which would involve spending the night at a local hospital.

Dr. T. told me not to worry. He was certain these tests would get to the root of my problem, and that there were treatments and medications that could help in either eventuality.

He was trying to reassure me, but I knew what I was facing. I knew that Alzheimer's is an incurable, fatal disease. [I later found out 35% of Americans don't know that Alzheimer's is fatal.][4] There are currently medications available that can slow the progress of the disease, but it can't be reversed. And it can't be stopped. And it can't be cured.

Yes, I know there are medications for Alzheimer's. Yes, I know there are many steps one can take, diet, exercise, and other techniques, to help cope, and in some cases maybe even slow the progression of the disease.

But I also know that if, in point of fact, I do indeed have Alzheimer's disease, one day it is going to kill me—if some other disease Alzheimer's helps along doesn't kill me first.

Friday, June 15, 2012

Today was my first appointment with Dr. W., my neurologist. When I called to make an appointment I was told the next available appointment was in August. I told this to Dr. T., and he called to let them know I could not wait. Today's appointment was scheduled soon after.

Dr. W. explained to me that she was an Alzheimer's specialist. She asked me to go over the issues that had caused me to go to Dr.T. with my concerns.

Then she began asking me a series of questions, the first of which was, "Can you name the President of the United States?" But from there things got a good deal more complicated. She grilled me orally for fifteen minutes or so, having me try to repeat different series of words and numbers in the same order she said them. Then she would ask me to remember a phrase. She'd go on to something else, and come back a short while later to see if I could still repeat the phrase correctly.

Dr. W. sat me down with a test booklet. I was to complete the booklet as quickly as possible without rushing, (Is that an oxymoron?), and let her nurse know when I was finished.

So I began. There were a variety of problems, like figuring out what came next in a series of numbers. There were questions that asked me to give the common factor in a group of objects. There were some word problems as well: "Alice is 4 years younger than Barbara and 2 years older than Clara. If Clara is 10, how old are the other two girls?"

I finished the test and the nurse took it to Dr. W. When the doctor came in about fifteen minutes later, she told me the results of her examination had been inconclusive as to Alzheimer's. She didn't have enough information to make a call either way.

Dr. W. said she was scheduling me for an intensive all day testing session that would definitively determine if I had Alzheimer's. Due to its length and complexity, and the personnel needed to conduct the testing session, there would be a very substantial wait before could be scheduled. They would schedule me as soon as possible and inform me of the date.

Monday, July 2, 2012

I haven't written in this diary for a couple of weeks now. The entire subject of Alzheimer's, and especially the uncertainty of not knowing, was really starting to get to me. I was having trouble sleeping. And I was having trouble concentrating. My thoughts kept returning to "what if." What if I *do* have it? What if I can no longer maintain my independence? What if I'm not able to finish the book I'm writing right now? How long do I have? These unanswerable questions swirled in my head night and day. So I decided the best thing to do was to just try to put it out of my mind for a while.

Dr. W's office had called to let me know the soonest they could schedule me for the all day Alzheimer's testing would be October 9th. Great. I'm going to be in this limbo of not knowing for another three months. I asked if there was any way they could make the test sooner, but they could not. This test was an all-day session using the services of several doctors and technicians, all concentrated on just me. It took some fancy scheduling to pull all the needed pieces together. Not to mention the fact that there were so many other people ahead of me that also needed this test. They assured me they were scheduling me on the earliest possible date.

For some reason I started thinking about Mama today, thinking about when things started to go awry with her. There was the mixing up of names thing. Then I found out about the problem with her driving and getting lost. But my stepfather was still alive then, so he was the one who took her to doctors' visits and assisted her through the process of diagnosis.

Mama was pretty far along in the development of her Alzheimer's before she was properly diagnosed. Back when Mama started showing symptoms, Alzheimer's wasn't nearly as well known, or as much talked about, as it is today. In fact, so little was known or said about it that a lot of people I know thought the disease was called "Old Timers."

Since some degree of memory loss and other similar symptoms truly are natural for people as they grow older, and most people knew very little (if anything) about Alzheimer's when Mama's symptoms first appeared, no mental alarms went off for us. In those days I think a lot of older people were not diagnosed until the disease had progressed much farther than is the norm for diagnosis today.

I know in my mother's case that was certainly true. Her memory lapses had been going on for years before someone in our family finally said, "Hey, I know she's getting older, but this is getting intense." I guess we really hadn't made a point of discussing what was happening with Mama's doctor until about that point.

Once her doctor was put on board, he set her up for testing, and sure enough, the verdict came back: Alzheimer's. So many people in my family have had the big A (as I am coming to think of it), but my mother was one of the first. And since long life also runs in my mother's family, the problem was exacerbated. My grandma lived to be 101. My mom passed away when she was 92. My brother is 74, and his Alzheimer's has gotten quite severe. [My brother passed away in 2014.]

So since my relatives were extremely elderly, and back then Alzheimer's was virtually unknown, a lot of people, including my folks, didn't get an early diagnosis. Which is a shame.   Although there is no cure for Alzheimer's there are measures and medications that can help, in some cases even retarding (although not *stopping*) the progression of the disease.

Wednesday, July 18, 2012

I had a mild stroke in February 2011. I was blessed in that Tiffani got me to the hospital immediately, and I was able to receive the clot-busting drug t-PA (tissue plasminogen activator) well within the recommended three-hour time frame. When I first arrived at the hospital I was having problems with my memory, and my speech was slurred and garbled. But after a four-day hospital stay the only remaining sign of the stroke was a tendency to stutter a bit on occasion, which in time all but went away.

I realized I had dodged a bullet. But for the grace of God and quality medical care, I could have been a goner. For the first time in my life, I truly felt my mortality. I sat down then and completed a bucket list. Things I wanted to do while there was still time.

I did accomplish one major thing on the list. I had lost touch with my father's family. My Dad's family was just the opposite of my mother's. They tended to die young. Both my paternal grandparents died before I was born. My father died when I was only three. Although he had many siblings, they had all died before I reached adulthood.

The only paternal relatives I knew of were two cousins, siblings. Their father and my father were brothers. After many years of not knowing each other's whereabouts, we reconnected via the internet.

I wanted to have them and their children over for dinner but had never acted on it. The stroke was my impetus to finally do it. They drove in from Ohio, and we had a wonderful time.

But all the other items on my bucket list remained unfulfilled. As I waited for my verdict on the big A, I realized this was the time to put these other missions in motion, while I still could.

I had been a singer all my life, even using some early gigs to help pay my way through college. I had always wanted to record an album. Right about this time, a karaoke friend serendipitously told me about a recording engineer with very reasonable rates.

I met with Nate, the sound engineer. I've started recording my CD! Nate does a very professional presentation, with artwork on the CD itself, a great picture cover and full liner notes. The CD is a collection of smooth jazz standards, and I'm calling it "Singing in the Rayne."[My stage name.] Of course, the song "Singing in the Rain" is on the CD.

When the CD is complete and I distribute it to family and friends, I know they are going to wonder what prompted me to do it. Maybe one day I'll tell them.

Thursday, August 02, 2012

I'm diabetic. I have been for 15 years. As a diabetic, I have a glucometer and I have to check my glucose levels often.

The glucometer I use turns itself on when you insert a test strip. I inserted a test strip this morning but the glucometer did not turn on. My first thought was that the battery was dead. But the glucometer has another mode that allows the user to check past readings. This mode is initiated by pushing a button. I pushed the button and the meter came on and gave me past readings just fine. So I knew the problem was not the battery.

I looked at the expiration date on the bottle of test strips I was using. The date was June 2013, so that was not the problem; the strips were not expired.

I was about half way through this bottle of strips, having already used 25 or so of the 50 strips it originally contained. That indicted the strips were not themselves defective.

Still, I went to get a new bottle of strips, thinking if another batch of strips wouldn't work I had a bigger problem. That would mean that the meter itself was defective. I groaned at the thought of having to go through the process of getting a new meter.

I got a new bottle of strips and after checking to make sure they were not expired, I opened the bottle and pulled out a new strip. Just before I inserted the strip into the meter I realized the problem: I had been sticking the wrong end of the strip into the meter. I had been putting the end of the strip meant for the blood sample into the meter. Once I realized this and turned the strip around to the correct configuration the meter came on to test with no problem at all.

Tuesday, August 21, 2012

Today I had an appointment with Nate, my recording engineer, to have a picture taken for my CD's cover and as my new author profile picture. Nate is also a photographer; in fact, his recording studio is in the same building as his photography studio.

The location is some 25 miles from my house in a portion of town that I don't know well; actually, I don't know it at all. On my first visit there, to record some songs, I had my GPS and a MapQuest printout. On my second visit, also to record, I was able to find my way there without either one.

Today I was going for just the photo session. I didn't worry about directions since this was my third time there. I knew my way to the freeway, and I knew how to get to the studio once I exited the freeway.

But as I approached the part of town where the studio was, I suddenly realized I couldn't remember which freeway exit to take. I wound up taking the wrong one and found myself in a part of town I had never been in before, and I had no idea how to get back on track. I didn't bring my GPS with me since I didn't think I needed it. (This was before I had GPS on my cell phone.)

Fortunately, the studio is at the intersection of two major streets, and just by dumb luck, I stumbled upon one of the streets. I followed it, hoping I was going in the right direction and found the studio.

Monday, September 3, 2012

Today is Labor Day and many members of my family were meeting at my brother's home for a family barbecue. I'm trying to remember when I last saw my brother. I think it was a year ago at Mama's funeral. My brother is 12 years older than me, so he's in his 70s, and like our mother has very advanced Alzheimer's disease.

When I got to his home for the picnic almost all of my family was in the backyard. I talked with cousins and other relatives I hadn't seen for a long time, and after a while, I asked someone where my brother was since I didn't see him. They told me that he was in the house and that he wasn't planning to come outside. I went in to see him. He and my sister-in-law were sitting in their living room looking at a baseball game on television.

I chatted a bit with them both, well, actually more with my sister-in-law. My brother was so deeply involved with the baseball game he really wasn't a part of the conversation. After a bit my sister-in-law needed to tell one of their children something, so she left the room to go outside.

I watched the game with Roland for a while. After a bit, I said to him, "You know, yesterday was the one year anniversary of Mama's death."

He turned to me with a puzzled look and said, "Who?"

"Mama."

"Whose Mama?"

I realized then what the problem was, and I was so sorry for even bringing it up.

"*Our* mama, Roland," I said gently. "Remember?"

He looked at me like I was out of my mind, and said, "*Our* Mama? Our mama ain't dead."

I didn't know what to do. I didn't know what to say. Maybe this was better. Maybe this was his way of handling Mama's loss—and who's to say it isn't a better way?

While I was sitting there trying to come up with the right thing to say, he had lost interest in our conversation and gone back to closely watching the baseball game.

I told him I'd be back and left the room to find my sister-in-law. I found her outside with the barbecue crowd. I pulled her aside, and told her, "I'm so sorry, I made a really big mistake with Roland just now. I wasn't thinking and I didn't realize he might take it that way."

She looked at me with concern and asked, "What happened?"

"I was telling him that yesterday was the one-year anniversary of the day Mama died, and he didn't remember. He just looked at me and said, 'Mama ain't dead.' He didn't seem upset about it, but I feel terrible bringing the whole thing up."

She looked at me and sadly shook her head. "Don't worry about it, girl. In a half hour, he'll have forgotten all about it."

Sunday, September 23, 2012

I just realized I have lost the ability to multi-task. I used to be a master at it. When you're a working single Mom you have to be.

I've been wondering why it takes me so long to get things done now. It is partially because of unpredictable "down" time from illness, but the main reason is that I can't multi-task anymore.

I think I must have been in denial about this because now that I've faced it, I realize I haven't even been *trying* to multi-task for months. I guess at some point I subconsciously perceived the problem but refused to openly face it, until today.

Friday, September 28, 2012

This morning when I got up one of the first things I did, as usual, was to fix myself a pot of coffee. As I stood at the kitchen counter putting the Truvia and creamer in the cup, I get a weird feeling but dismiss it, because I see no basis for it.

I go into my office with the cup of coffee, and lo and behold, there sits another cup of coffee. I had already made myself a cup of coffee but did not remember that I had until I saw it sitting there.

Of late I am having more and more of what I am calling "What the hell did you do that for?" moments. Doing something and forgetting I did it, or doing it incorrectly when I've been doing it correctly for years, or not doing something but believing I had, and only later realizing I didn't.

Saturday, September 29, 2012

[Since 2003 I have owned and operated an online antique and collectible shop, "Raynetta's Romantiques."]

Lord help me. I just realized that since January 24, 2012, I have listed a beautiful pair of vintage Weiss earrings as a *brooch*!

I often take a description of an item from a past listing and modify it to fit the new item I'm posting. That is not unusual, but the fact that I didn't do the modification correctly, or catch the error in eight months' time is frightening. What else have I done incorrectly in my shop?

To date, 127 people have viewed this item. No wonder it hasn't sold. I sure wish somebody had been kind enough to drop me a note about it.

Sunday, September 30, 2012

More and more frequently I find myself thinking one word but writing another.

For instance, just now Doug [my significant other] told me he needed two more of my books for a co-worker. He's a male nurse. He works with a lot of women, and many of them like romance novels.

I was writing myself a sticky note as a reminder. I meant to write "2 books for Jane," but started off with "too." Yesterday I was trying to write the word "friends" and wrote the word "fries."

I'm going to try to keep track of when and how this happens.

Tuesday, October 9, 2012

Well, this is the long awaited day, the day I have my extensive neuropsychological testing. This is the testing my neurologist needs to determine if I have Alzheimer's— or not.

The testing will take all day. It was originally scheduled for 8:30 AM to 4:30 PM, but I got a call yesterday from the test center. They wanted to know if I could reschedule for another day due to some issues on their end. I told them I didn't want to do that since Tiffani had requested time off work months ago in order to go with me. They then said they could still see me on the 9th, but changed the time to 9:30 AM to 4 PM.

So here I am at 8:30, dressed and ready to go. I'm afraid, but I know this is a necessary step. If I do have Alzheimer's I know from what happened to my mother the sooner I start treatment and medication the better the odds they will perhaps retard the progress of the disease.

But I hate the fact that it will still be two more months before I can get the diagnosis. I was told it takes 6 six weeks for the results of the testing to be finalized. So I have an appointment with my neurologist for December 4th. We allowed ample time to be certain she would have the test results in hand.

So I'll just have to continue walking the tightrope until then, still not knowing, but I having no choice but to wait. And to pray.

Wednesday, October 10, 2012

The test yesterday went smoothly. The first part was an intensive interview with not one but two psychiatrists. Tiffani was there during that interview and gave the doctors her input as to my behavior and actions.

We talked about my history: my grandmother, mother, brother and some aunts having Alzheimer's. I told them about my stroke last year and about my car accident in December 2011. About my confusion and stuttering and difficulty finding words.

I was surprised when Tiffani told them about her sensing my confusion, and about me repeating myself and telling her things I had already told her but had forgotten I had told her. [In reading over this diary later, I realized she *had* told me about repeating myself, but at the point of this interview with the doctors I had forgotten that.]

This interview lasted about 2 hours. Both psychiatrists were professional but personable. They listened to me carefully and took tons of notes. They asked a multitude of questions to clarify things I said.

I went to lunch and the afternoon session was a long progression of tests. Some of the tests seemed really strange to me, like having me cross off "2s" and "7s" on a page filled with numbers and letters. There were about eight sections of this and I was timed on each section. Dr. Z (one of the psychiatrists) was timing me with a stopwatch and would tell me when to start and when to stop each section. I didn't finish any of the sections. I hope that's not a bad sign.

The other tests involved lists of words and how I could repeat those. I was tested on the meanings of words. I also had to duplicate patterns and shapes—duplicating drawings first while looking at the original, and after an interval, drawing it again from memory. And yes, I had to put round pegs—with a square side—into holes!

October 13, 2012

Have you ever worked with, or lived with, or been married to someone you could not trust? Not that they were deliberately trying to mislead you, but they were so unpredictable you did not know what to expect? That you didn't know which, if any, of the actions they took or statements they made you could rely on?

That's what's happening to me. Except that the person I can't trust anymore is myself. I can't rely on my memory because it might lie to me. I hide things from myself, not meaning to, but I put things down, and a minute later I can't remember where they are.

Monday, October 15, 2012

I keep track of my appointments and tasks using Microsoft Outlook. Today a task reminder popped up that referenced an email my daughter sent me three months ago. There was no action to take on it and I have no recollection of why I set this task. In fact, I have no memory of setting it in the first place.

Thursday, October 18, 2012

The problems I'm having with words and language are really playing hell with my career as a novelist.

I never took formal typing lessons (maybe I should). After all these years of being a professional writer I type fairly fast, but since I don't "touch type," I watch the keyboard and not the computer screen.

Today I wanted to type the sentence "There is a tiny nick in the card." When I looked up at the screen I had typed "The is a tiny nic in the yard."

When I mistype a word it seems to rarely be just a random typo. The mistyped word is always another word: "the" for "there" or "yard" for "card," for instance. I think in the above example I typed "nic" for "nick" because I just finished working on a novel that had a character named "Ric," spelled that way rather than the more common "Rick."

What makes this an ultra pain in the ass for a writer is that spell check will not catch this. Spell check is geared to catch misspelled words. If I use the wrong word, but use something that is indeed itself a word, spell check won't catch it unless it causes a grammatical error. So I'm having to proof read my work with an extra fine tooth comb to catch these types of errors.

I find this happens when I speak, as well. I'll mean to say "robust" and what comes out is "robot." This is really scary because most of the time I don't realize I've done it. If I'm talking to somebody close to me like my man or my daughter, they will point it out to me. But if I'm talking to a stranger or someone I don't know well they usually won't.

I'm sensitive to this problem now. Sometimes when I'm talking to someone a strange look will cross their face while I'm speaking. I've gotten to the point now where I just ask them if I said something that didn't make sense. Sometimes they'll say yes and tell me what it was.

But sometimes they'll say, "Oh, no, you didn't say anything wrong," but they'll say it in a way that lets me know I did. They didn't want to say so either out of fear of offending me or because they just plain didn't want to be bothered.

Friday, October 19, 2012

Today's faux pas:

While driving down Telegraph road, I wanted to take I-696 east to go home. I instead took I-696 west, which took me a total of about 10 miles out of my way.

The point where I got on the freeway is less than 5 minutes from my house. I have been living in this house for 16 years and must have taken that route home literally hundreds of times. But for some unknown reason, today my demon told me to take it in the wrong direction.

When I finally got home I made myself a pot of coffee. The only problem was I forgot to put water in the coffee maker. So when I went back 10 minutes later to get my coffee, all I found was a hot, but empty, pot.

Also this week I totally screwed up editing my most recent book by using the wrong name for a character throughout the second half of the book.

Monday, October 22, 2012

[I had great difficulty coping with my mother's death, so
Dr. T. suggested I get grief counseling.]

I had an appointment with my counselor today. We talked
about the Alzheimer situation. She is of the option that the
testing I had earlier this month still may not be conclusive.
She feels the neurologist, even with those test results,
possibly will still not be able to definitively say yea or nay
on the Alzheimer's.

I'm certainly not eager to be diagnosed with the big A, but
neither am I eager to walk around between heaven and hell,
not knowing for another year. Which is what my counselor
said would happen if they can't make a call on it now.
They would just schedule me to take the mega test again in
a year.

Great.

Friday, October 26, 2012

The "different word" merry-go-round continues. I just
wrote "get back" instead of "get by" in an internet post.
Once again, these glitches are so treacherous because the
wrong word is still a word, so spell check won't catch it.
It's hell when the person sabotaging your work is you.

Tuesday, October 30, 2012

My neurologist's office called to switch my appointment from December 4 to November 30. Good. Just that much earlier that I will (hopefully) have the verdict!

Wednesday, October 31, 2012

Trick or Treat!

Well, unfortunately for me, it's been more tricks than treats lately. As well as the continuing word mix-up problem, now I seem to be having problems with capital letters! I am routinely and frequently omitting capital letters, even when typing my own name!

It is so tough not sharing what is going on with me with friends and family. I've made so many glaring boo-boos in front of some of my friends, but I'm determined not to tell them about the possible Alzheimer's. I don't want them feeling sorry for me. I don't want to talk about it. Or maybe I just don't want to acknowledge it. I don't know.

After I get the diagnosis, if I do have the big A, I'll have to make a decision then on when and what to tell people. But I'm not even going to entertain that issue until then.

Am I afraid? Yes, I have to admit I am. This is worse than the time I had a lump in my breast. It was about 10 days after I saw my regular doctor before I could get an appointment with the surgeon. It would have been months, but Dr. T (bless him!) called and told them I couldn't wait. Then, after I saw the surgeon, it was about a month before they could arrange the surgery. Then it was two weeks after the surgery before I got the results of the lab tests. Thank God, the tumor was not malignant.

I thought waiting for that diagnosis was hard, but this waiting is somehow so much harder. I'm not sure why.

No, I take that back. I do know why. This is harder because a diagnosis of breast cancer would have left me some hope. I would have been diagnosed early after the discovery of the lump. That statistically would have meant my chances of the cancer not being fatal would have been good.

But if I have Alzheimer's there essentially is no hope. There is no cure. All I can hope for is to use medicine and other means to retard the progress of the disease as much as possible. But if I have it I'll have it until the day I die. And I'm scared to death that my brain will die before my body does.

Word mix-ups: These are the words I've mixed up just in typing this short entry:

that for than
own for our
seem for even
then for them
let for left
changes for chances
jut for just

Thursday, November 01, 2012

One of my customers from my online antique shop emailed me this morning. I have a Fenton vase for sale in my shop. The price was showing as $4,539.00. The customer emailed me asking "Is this price correct?"

He was very tactful in bringing this boo-boo to my attention. I'm sure he knew the price was *way* out of line for the vase.

What happened was I had originally priced the vase at $45.00. When it didn't sell at that price I went in to lower it to a sale price of $39.00.

I sent him a thank you note. If he hadn't brought it to my attention I may not have caught it for months, if at all. As well as the vase not selling, it would have sat there in my shop making me look uninformed and/or careless and/or ridiculously greedy as an antique dealer.

Friday, November 30, 2012

Well, today is the day. I'm apprehensive and scared. I didn't realize just how scared I was until I woke up this morning.

This is a chain of events that began almost a year ago, on December 18, 2011, when I had my car accident.

I want to know the answer. I've been tormented all these months not knowing. And yet… While unknowing I at least had the luxury of saying to myself, "Maybe I *don't* have it."

But after today I won't have that comfort. I will have either the joy of *knowing* I don't have it or the despair of *knowing* I do. No middle ground. All the marbles are bet on this one roll of the dice. Either I have Alzheimer's—or I do not. I'm finally going to know.

I'm leaving for the doctor's office now. I'm going to say a prayer before I go.

Epilogue

Thank God, I do not have Alzheimer's. At least, not yet.

Dr. W. told me the mega test left no doubt. I do not at this
point have Alzheimer's. But she did emphasize the "at this
point." She told me with the combination of my age, my
present medical condition, and my inauspicious family
history, I was high risk for developing Alzheimer's as the
years progressed.

She recommended I have an appointment with her every
two years as a follow-up. And I should, of course, come in
immediately if I felt my situation had changed for the
worse.

So it turned out that my problems were being caused by
Dr.T.'s other suspect, sleep apnea.

I was to undergo the sleep apnea screening at the same time
I was being evaluated for Alzheimer's. But there was an
appointment I had waited a long time for that the sleep
clinic had to cancel. One of the nurses there told me they
were experiencing an extreme, although temporary, staffing
shortage.

I didn't wind up having my sleep study until March 2013.
That test was a doozy as well. I had more wires stuck to
me than a time bomb. And they had the nerve to expect me
to sleep that way!

But I did finally fall asleep. The sleep clinic staff
determined I woke up 120 times an hour, although the sleep
disruptions were so brief I couldn't consciously detect
them. My problems were not caused by deterioration of
my brain. The problems were caused by my brain being

starved for oxygen, due to my continuously interrupted sleep.

I now have to sleep wearing a face mask attached to a CPAP (Continuous Positive Airway Pressure) machine. It can be awkward and was at first somewhat uncomfortable, but I'm used to it now.

My symptoms began to clear up almost immediately. It was unbelievable that I could improve so much so quickly.

So that's my story. Although I don't have Alzheimer's (yet), I'm on a mission to increase Alzheimer's awareness and Alzheimer's research.

Many experts are now using the term "Alzheimer's Tsunami."

"In most of the world, the increasing prevalence of Alzheimer's disease is building up slowly, just like a tsunami far out in the midst of the ocean....When it hits, the tsunami will cause havoc and destruction, and will probably do so suddenly. The longer we wait the more intense and more devastating the effects will be. We must, therefore, plan ahead for the coming of this irresistible onslaught of an Alzheimer's tsunami."[5]

As I stated at the beginning of this journal, it was not originally intended for publication. But now that it is available, I hope it helps someone who is going through the valley of the shadow of Alzheimer's diagnosis.

Bibliography

1. DeMarco, Bob. "100 Million Adults Touched by Alzheimer's Disease." Alzheimer's Reading Room. http://www.alzheimersreadingroom.com/2009/05/100-million-adults-touched-by.html Accessed March 28, 2013.

2. Ayers, Mike. " Oscars 2015: The Story Behind Glen Campbell's 'I'm Not Gonna Miss You'" The Wall Street Journal. http://blogs.wsj.com/speakeasy/2015/02/19/oscars-2015-the-story-behind-glen-campbells-im-not-gonna-miss-you/ Accessed Feb. 19, 2015

3. Wikipedia, the free encyclopedia http://en.wikipedia.org/wiki/Diary

4. Alzheimer Europe.org. "Public Knowledge of Alzheimer's Disease [Survey] http://www.alzheimer-europe.org/Research/Value-of-Knowing/Public-knowledge-of-Alzheimer-s-disease Accessed April 17, 2013

5. Wallack, Max. "The Coming Alzheimer's Tsunami" The Alzheimer's Reading Room http://www.alzheimersreadingroom.com/2013/04/the-coming-alzheimers-tsunami.html

Accessed July 14, 2014

Alzheimer's Resources Online

The Alzheimer's Association

http://www.alz.org/alzheimers_disease_causes_risk_factors
.asp

Alzheimers.net

http://www.alzheimers.net/stages-of-alzheimers-disease /

Alzheimer's Reading Room

https://plus.google.com/+Alzheimersreadingroom1/posts

The Fisher Center Foundation for Alzheimer's Research

http://www.alzinfo.org/about /

The Mayo Clinic: Alzheimer's Disease

http://www.mayoclinic.org/diseases-conditions/alzheimers-
disease/basics/definition/con-20023871

WebMD: Alzheimer's Disease Health Center

http://www.webmd.com/alzheimers/guide/treatment-
overview

Raynetta Manees' Alzheimer's Board on Pinterest

https://www.pinterest.com/raynettamanees/alzheimers-
disease/

OTHER BOOKS BY RAYNETTA MANEES

All For Love
(The SuperStar Series: Book One)
Available in Kindle Nook Paperback

All For Love: The SuperStar
(The SuperStar Series: Book Two)
Available in Kindle Nook Paperback

Wishing On A Star
Available in Kindle Nook Paperback

All The Way Home
Available in Kindle Nook Paperback

Fantasy
Available in Kindle Nook Paperback

Follow Your Heart
Available in Kindle Nook Paperback

Classic Paperback Books

All For Love
released September 1996, ISBN 0-7860-0309-X
rated 5 stars on both Amazon and B&N

Wishing On A Star
released August 1997, ISBN 0-7860-0423-1
rated 4 ½ stars Amazon   5 stars B&N

Follow Your Heart
released September 1998 ISBN 0-7860-0560-2
rated 5 stars on both Amazon and B&N

Fantasy
released August 1999 ISBN 1-58314-030-1
rated 5 stars on both Amazon and B&N

Heart Of The Matter
Heart of the Matter, released January 2002 ISBN 1-58314-262-2
rated 5 stars Amazon   Not yet rated on B&N

A Mother's Touch
A three author anthology containing Raynetta Manees' novella,
"All The Way Home"
released May 1999 ISBN 1-58314-015-8
Rated 5 stars on both Amazon and B&N

ABOUT THE AUTHOR

Raynetta Manees is a best-selling, award-winning author. Her books are in both digital and print editions and she is traditionally published and self-published. She's done it all! She has written several five-star Black romance novels as well as a non-fiction book about #Alzheimer's. All Raynetta's books are on Amazon and B&N.

Her landmark first-person novel, **All For Love**, first released in 1996, is now considered a Black romance classic. An updated e-book edition of the novel was released in 2013. This book is now Book One of *The SuperStar Series.*

September 2016 marked Raynetta's 20th anniversary as an author. She celebrated this milestone with the release of Book Two of *The SuperStar Series*, **All For Love: The Superstar** in Sept 2016. The book is a finalist for the 2017 Emma Award for the Best Contemporary Romance of the year. The Emma is the premier award for black authors of romance.

Raynetta is the very first recipient of the Award of Excellence from RomanceInColor.com for her novel **Follow Your Heart.**

She is currently working on Book Three of *The SuperStar Series*, **All For Love: The Superstar's Daughter**, which will be released in 2018.

Raynetta's author page on Amazon.com is www.amazon.com/author/raynettamanees

All of Raynetta's books are rated four/five stars by readers on Amazon.com and BN.com (Barnes and Noble).

Raynetta Manees is a graduate of Wayne State University, with a degree in Mass Communications. She retired as a Federal government executive administrator after a 28-year career. Raynetta now writes full-time. Her love of the media arts is reflected in her novels, whose characters are involved in some aspect of entertainment/media.

Raynetta has been a solo vocalist since childhood. Her stage name is "Rayne," and her first CD, "Singing in the Rayne," a collection of smooth jazz vocals, was released in December 2012.

The author is an accomplished actress who has appeared in numerous stage productions and in TV and radio commercials. As an on-air radio personality, she was known as "Shalimar Brown, the baddest girl in town" on AM 1180 WXLA.

Raynetta stepped away from her career as a notable romance novelist in June 2015 to pen her first non-fiction work, **My Alzheimer's Diary.** The book explores Alzheimer's effect on her family and her own journey of diagnosis.

Raynetta welcomes your comments at her website www.RManees.com. She can also be reached via email at RManees@aol.com (Please show "Reader" and your name in the subject line.)

You may also reach Raynetta via:
Facebook: Raynetta Manees, Author
Twitter: @raynettaman,
Pinterest: Raynetta Manees Author on Pinterest
Instagram: ms.manees
Mail: P.O. Box 3203, Southfield, MI 48037
Goodreads Author Page:
goodreads.com/author/show/21931.Raynetta_Manees